# OVERCOMING ALLERGIES

## The Ultimate Guide With Practical Strategies For Winning Over Allergies

**Walker I. Eastman**

# TABLE OF CONTENT

# INTRODUCTION

I used to be a prisoner of my own body, bound in the merciless grasp of allergies. Every season brought a wave of misery, leaving me sneezing, itching, and gasping for air. Life seemed like a never-ending war against phantom opponents.

But then, one day, I came onto a glimpse of optimism. Through several trials and mistakes, I found a road to release from the shackles of allergies. The remedies I uncovered were the core crux of this book, "Allergies Uncovered: Practical Strategies for Winning Over Allergies."

Within these pages lay the answers that altered my life. I devoted my heart and soul into uncovering the secrets of allergies, armed myself with information and practical methods to battle their unrelenting onslaught. From comprehending the numerous sorts of allergies to refuting popular misunderstandings, I leave no stone untouched.

I provide the key to uncovering the hidden causes of allergies, helping you discover your triggers, and traverse the maze of allergy testing procedures. Together, we will discover the hidden reasons that intensify your symptoms, allowing you to take ownership of your health.

But this book is not only about understanding allergies; it's about finding the light at the end of the tunnel. I offer realistic techniques to overcome allergies, from effective management tactics and lifestyle tweaks to boosting your immune system. These answers have altered my life, and now they can improve yours too.

Dear reader, I encourage you to read on. Journey with me as we begin on a search for liberation from the bonds of allergies. This is your opportunity to recover your life, to breathe deeply without fear, and to embrace a future where allergies no longer keep you prisoner.

Don't settle for a life riddled with continual sneezing, itching, and pain. Together, let us learn the secrets, embrace the practical techniques, and release the power to fight allergies. It's time to open the pages, absorb the wisdom inside, and unlock the door to a life free from the torture of allergies.

The trip awaits. Will you join me?

# CHAPTER 1

## BOOK OVERVIEW

Welcome to "Overcoming Allergies," a thorough handbook that will enable you to beat allergies and restore control of your life. In this book, we will discuss practical tactics and helpful insights to help you understand and conquer allergies efficiently.

Whether you're coping with seasonal allergies, food allergies, or any other sort, the knowledge and practices presented here will give you with the skills you need to survive. Let's go on this trip together.

Allergies affect millions of individuals worldwide, and their effect may vary from minor discomfort to serious health issues. This book is meant to address the major issues experienced by allergy patients, debunk misunderstandings, and equip you with a practical path to confront allergies head-on.

In the following chapters, we will dig into the basic features of allergies, beginning with a clear grasp of what allergies actually are and the common forms you may face. We will clarify frequent myths and misunderstandings about allergies, enabling you to have a more realistic view on this widespread health condition.

Understanding allergies is only the beginning. To successfully conquer them, it is vital to discover their core causes. Chapter 3 will assist you through the process of determining allergy triggers particular to your condition. By learning how to detect the things that trigger off your symptoms, you may take proactive actions to reduce exposure and manage your allergies more successfully.

Allergy testing is a helpful tool in the process toward identifying your triggers. In Chapter 3, we will study several testing procedures, including skin prick tests and blood tests, giving you with insights into their merits and limits. Armed with this information, you may work together with healthcare experts to acquire accurate findings and make educated choices about treating your allergies.

But what about hidden allergy culprits? In Chapter 3, we will throw light on lesser-known triggers and variables that lead to allergies. Sometimes, allergies might be induced by cross-reactivity or unusual compounds that may not be immediately visible. By finding these hidden allergy factors, you may widen your awareness and take appropriate steps to prevent exposure.

Chapter 4 will present a practical approach to conquering allergies. We will review successful allergy treatment methods that involve a variety of alternatives, including drugs for symptom alleviation, allergen avoidance approaches, and preventative measures. Additionally, we will dig into lifestyle improvements that may considerably ease allergy symptoms. From building an allergy-friendly atmosphere at home to managing allergies in diverse contexts like work, school, or while vacation, you will receive useful insights and effective recommendations.

Moreover, we shall examine the necessity of boosting your immune system in Chapter 4. A healthy immune system may help decrease the severity of allergy responses and enhance your general well-being. By adding aspects such as diet, exercise, stress management, and quality sleep, you may strengthen your body's natural defenses against allergens and enhance your resilience.

In Chapter 5, we will complete our trip with a recap of the important concepts explored throughout the book. We will highlight the need of perseverance, patience, and customisation in finding the optimal technique for treating your allergies. Remember, everyone's allergy experience is unique, and it may take time to find the tactics that work best for you.

Finally, the appendix gives extra tools and information to help you on your allergy-fighting adventure. You will discover references to trustworthy organizations, glossaries of allergy-related words, and suggested reading resources for additional investigation.

Now that we have established the backdrop, let's go into Chapter 2, where we will obtain a better knowledge of allergies by analyzing what they are and the common varieties that exist. By creating a firm foundation of information, you will be well-equipped to take the required measures towards winning over allergies.

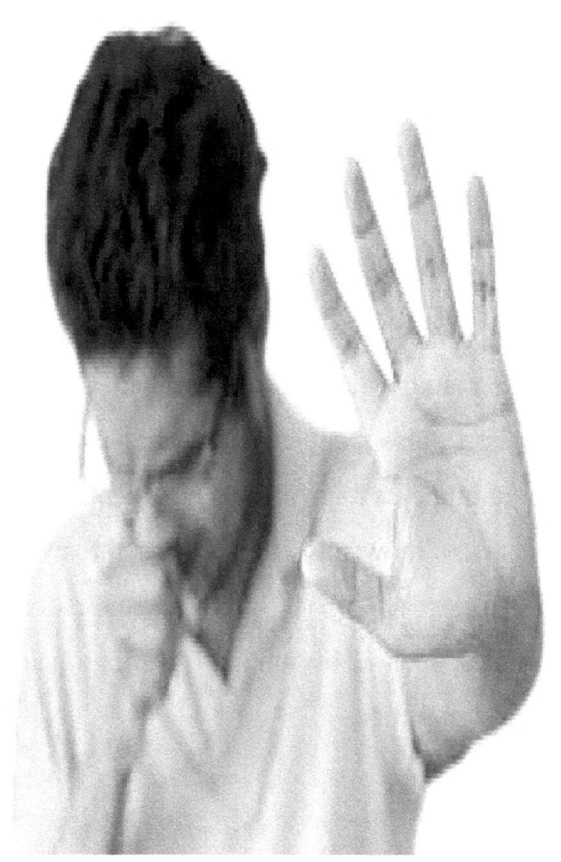

# CHAPTER 2

# UNDERSTANDING ALLERGIES

### What Are Allergies?

Allergies are the result of an overactive immune system reacting to substances that are typically harmless to most people. When you have an allergy, your immune system mistakenly identifies certain substances, known as allergens, as threats to your body. In reaction, it produces a cascade of molecules, such as histamines, creating a variety of allergic symptoms.

## Common Types of Allergies

Allergies may show in numerous ways, and identifying the precise kind you're dealing with is vital for successful treatment. Here are some typical forms of allergies:

## Respiratory Allergies

**<u>Hay Fever (Allergic Rhinitis)</u>**: Symptoms include sneezing, congestion, runny nose, and itchy/watery eyes. This form of allergy is commonly provoked by pollen, dust mites, or pet dander.

**<u>Asthma</u>:** Allergic asthma is induced by particular allergens, leading to inflammation and constriction of the airways, resulting in breathing problems, coughing, and wheezing.

## Food Allergies

Common food allergies include allergies to peanuts, tree nuts, shellfish, eggs, milk, wheat, and soy. Ingesting even little quantities of these allergens may elicit a variety of symptoms, from moderate responses like hives and stomach difficulties to severe anaphylaxis.

## Skin Allergies

**Contact Dermatitis:** This type of allergy occurs when the skin comes into contact with an allergen, leading to redness, itching, and sometimes blisters. Common culprits include certain metals (e.g., nickel), latex, and specific chemicals.

**Insect Sting Allergies:** Some people may experience severe allergic responses to insect stings, such as those from bees, wasps, or fire ants. These responses might vary from regional swelling and discomfort to systemic reactions that impact the entire body.

# Debunking Allergy Misconceptions

There are various misunderstandings about allergies that might obscure our awareness. Let's dispel some of these popular misconceptions:

## Allergies Are Merely A Minor Annoyance

Allergies may greatly damage your quality of life, creating chronic discomfort, limiting sleep, and hampering everyday activities. They should not be discounted as trivial inconveniences.

## Allergies Only Arise At Particular Seasons

While seasonal allergies are frequent, many allergens, such as pet dander, dust mites, and certain foods, may provoke allergies year-round.

## Allergies May Be Outgrown

While some children may outgrow particular allergies, many allergies linger until adulthood. It's crucial to manage allergies proactively and not expect they will fade with time.

## Allergies Are Not Major Health Conditions

Allergies may vary from moderate to severe, and in rare situations, they can be life-threatening, such as in cases of anaphylaxis. It is vital to take allergies seriously and seek proper treatment.

By debunking these misunderstandings, we may create a more realistic awareness of allergies and their influence on our lives. In the following chapter, we will go further into finding the fundamental causes of allergies, beginning with identifying allergy triggers that impact each person individually.

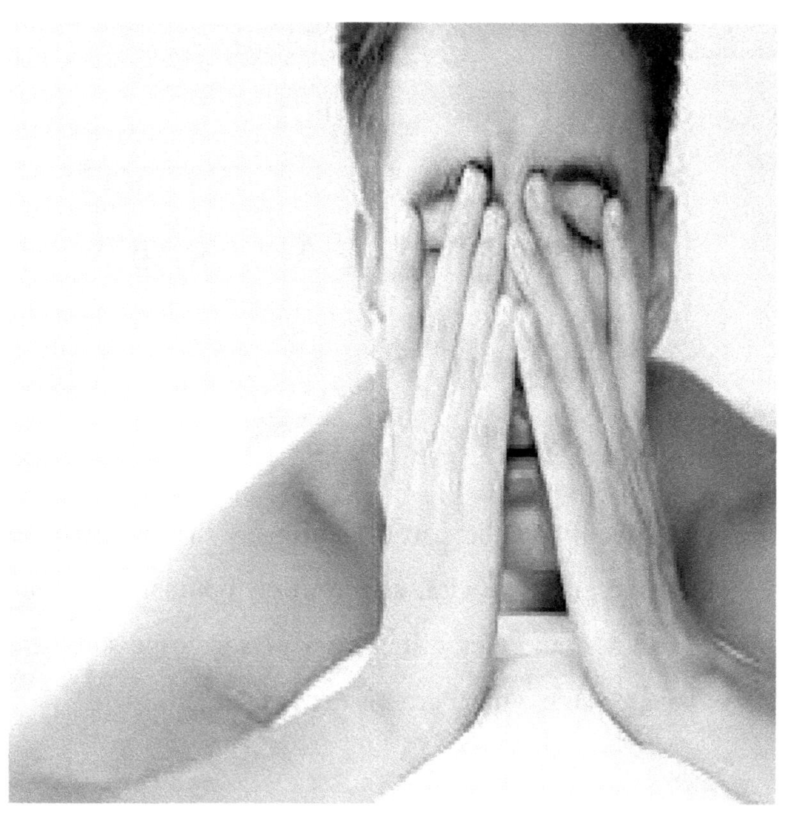

# CHAPTER 3

# UNCOVERING THE ROOT CAUSES OF ALLERGIES

## *Identifying Allergy Triggers*

Identifying the particular triggers that set off your allergies is a vital step towards optimal treatment. While allergies differ from person to person, here are some typical groups to consider:

## Environmental Allergens

**Pollen:** Different species of plants generate pollen, and exposure to particular pollens may elicit seasonal allergies.

**<u>Dust Mites:</u>** Microscopic creatures present in home dust, especially in bedding, upholstery, and carpets, may provoke allergic responses.

**<u>Pet Dander:</u>** Proteins contained in pet saliva, urine, and dander (dead skin flakes) may provoke allergies in sensitive persons.

## Food Allergens

Common allergic foods include peanuts, tree nuts, shellfish, fish, eggs, milk, wheat, soy, and some fruits and vegetables. Keeping a meal diary and documenting any unpleasant responses might help discover dietary triggers.

## Insect Allergens

Stings or bites from insects like bees, wasps, hornets, fire ants, or mosquitoes may provoke allergic responses in sensitive people.

## Allergy Testing Methods

If you're confused about your particular allergies, allergy testing might give helpful information. Here are two typical approaches used:

### Skin Prick Test

This test includes putting tiny quantities of allergens on your skin, generally on your forearm or back, and then pricking or scratching the skin to enable the allergen to enter. If you are allergic to a certain chemical, you'll acquire a little raised bump at the test location.

### Blood Tests

Blood tests, such as the particular IgE (Immunoglobulin E) test, evaluate the amount of allergen-specific antibodies in your blood. This test may assist identify possible allergies, particularly when skin prick testing are equivocal or not practicable.

# Medications

Certain medicines, such as antibiotics, nonsteroidal anti-inflammatory drugs (NSAIDs), and even over-the-counter pain treatments like aspirin, may induce adverse responses in certain people.

# Hidden Allergy Culprits

Sometimes, allergies might have underlying causes that are not immediately evident. Consider the following things that may lead to allergies:

### Cross-Reactivity

Cross-reactivity happens when your immune system responds to a chemical because it resembles another allergy. For example, if you have a pollen allergy, you may suffer cross-reactivity with some fruits or vegetables that contain comparable proteins.

## **Uncommon Triggers**

Allergies may be induced by less common items, such as particular spices, food additives, or chemicals in personal care products. Being aware of these less-obvious triggers might help you make educated decisions and prevent possible allergic responses.

By unraveling the fundamental causes of your allergies via trigger identification and testing, you may acquire a deeper knowledge of what you need to avoid or manage. Armed with this information, you'll be more able to take proactive efforts towards conquering your allergies.

In the following chapter, we will cover practical approaches to conquer allergies, including allergy management tactics, lifestyle improvements for allergy relief, and methods to build your immune system. Let's continue our path toward winning over allergies.

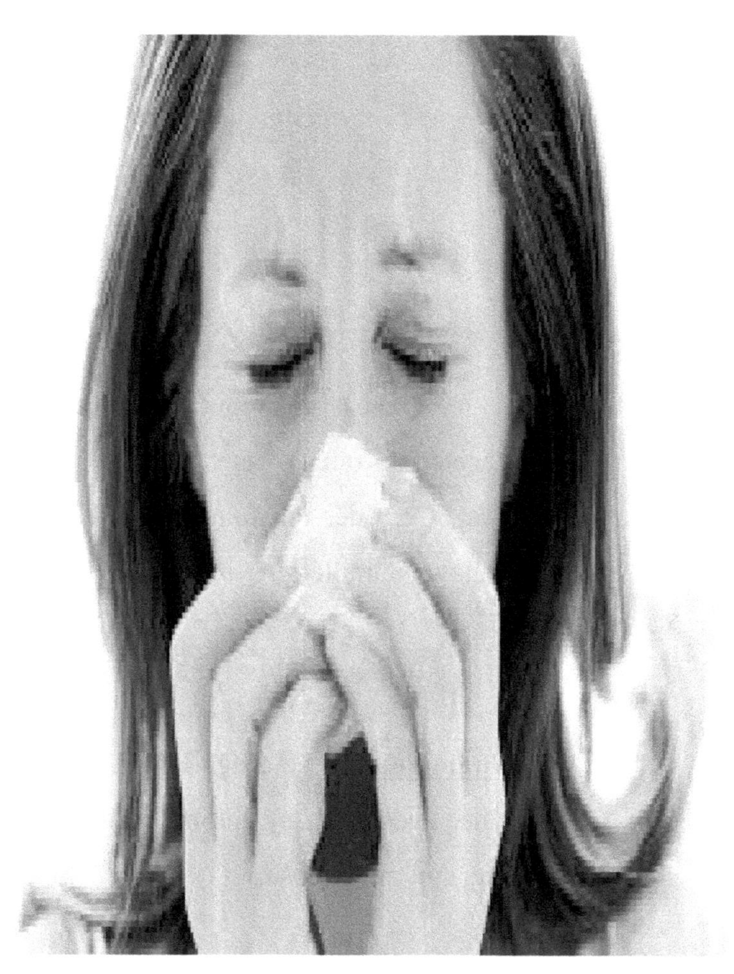

# CHAPTER 4

# PRACTICAL STEPS TO OVERCOME ALLERGIES

## *Allergy Management Strategies*

When it comes to controlling allergies, a multi-faceted strategy is generally the most beneficial. Consider the following ways to reduce and regulate your allergy symptoms:

## Medications

**Antihistamines:** These drugs inhibit the effects of histamine, decreasing symptoms including itching, sneezing, and runny nose.

**Nasal Sprays:** Corticosteroid nasal sprays assist decrease inflammation and congestion in the nasal passages.

**<u>Eye Drops:</u>** Specialized eye drops may ease itchy, red, and watery eyes caused by allergies.

**<u>Epinephrine Autoinjector:</u>** If you have a severe allergy, such as a food or insect sting allergy, carrying an epinephrine autoinjector may be life-saving in case of an anaphylactic response.

**<u>Allergen Avoidance:</u>**

Identify and limit exposure to your particular allergies. For example, use dust mite-proof coverings for bedding, keep dogs out of bedrooms, and routinely clean your living areas to avoid allergy collection.

## **Allergy-Proof Your Environment:**

Create an allergen-friendly atmosphere at home by utilizing high-efficiency particulate air (HEPA) filters, keeping windows closed during high pollen seasons, and maintaining adequate indoor air quality.

## **Allergy Immunotherapy:**

Allergy injections (subcutaneous immunotherapy) or sublingual immunotherapy (under-the-tongue tablets or drops) might be prescribed by allergists for long-term treatment, progressively desensitizing your immune system to certain allergens.

Lifestyle Adjustments for Allergy Relief

In addition to medical treatments, adopting some lifestyle improvements may help lessen allergy symptoms and enhance your general well-being:

### Maintain a Healthy Diet:

A balanced diet rich in fruits, vegetables, and whole grains may assist strengthen your immune system. Some studies show that omega-3 fatty acids, present in fish and flaxseed, may have anti-inflammatory qualities that might aid allergy patients.

### Keep Indoor Air Clean:

Routinely clean carpets, remove dust routinely, and use air purifiers to decrease interior allergies. Consider using a dehumidifier to reduce mold development in moist locations.

### Manage Stress:

Stress might increase allergy symptoms. Practice stress management strategies such as deep breathing exercises, meditation, or participating in activities you like to help lower stress levels.

### Exercise Wisely:

Engage in regular exercise to increase your general health and build your immune system. However, be aware of exercising outside during high pollen seasons, and consider indoor activities on days when allergen levels are high.

## Strengthening The Immune System

A healthy immune system may play a significant role in minimizing the severity of allergic responses. Consider the following immune-strengthening practices:

### Balanced Nutrition:

Consume a diet rich in vitamins, minerals, and antioxidants to help your immune system. Incorporate items like citrus fruits, leafy greens, nuts, and seeds into your meals.

## Regular Exercise:

Engage in moderate activity, such as brisk walking or cycling, to increase your general health and immunological function. Aim for at least 30 minutes of activity most days of the week.

## Quality Sleep:

Prioritize adequate and restful sleep, since it plays a critical role in immune system functioning and general well-being. Establish a regular sleep regimen and establish a pleasant sleep environment.

## Stress Management:

Chronic stress may impair the immune system. Practice stress-reducing practices such as meditation, yoga, or indulging in activities that offer you pleasure.

By taking these practical methods, you may greatly lessen the burden of allergies on your everyday life. Remember, everyone's allergies are unique, so it may take some trial and error to discover the tactics that work best for you.

In the last chapter, we will end our examination of allergens and highlight the major insights from this book. Let's go ahead on your road to conquer allergies and attain a better quality of life.

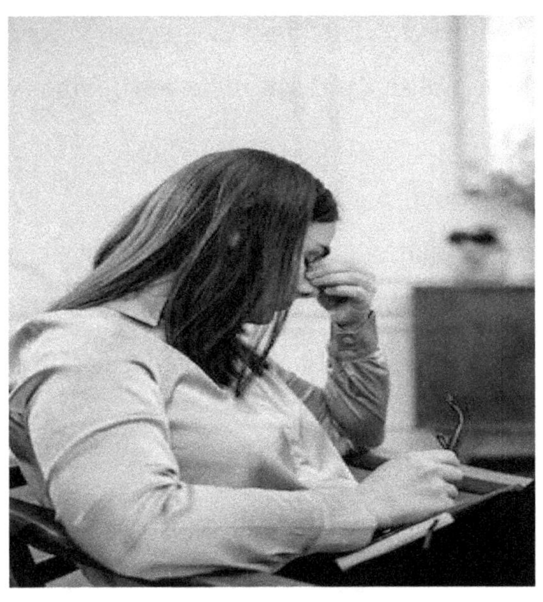

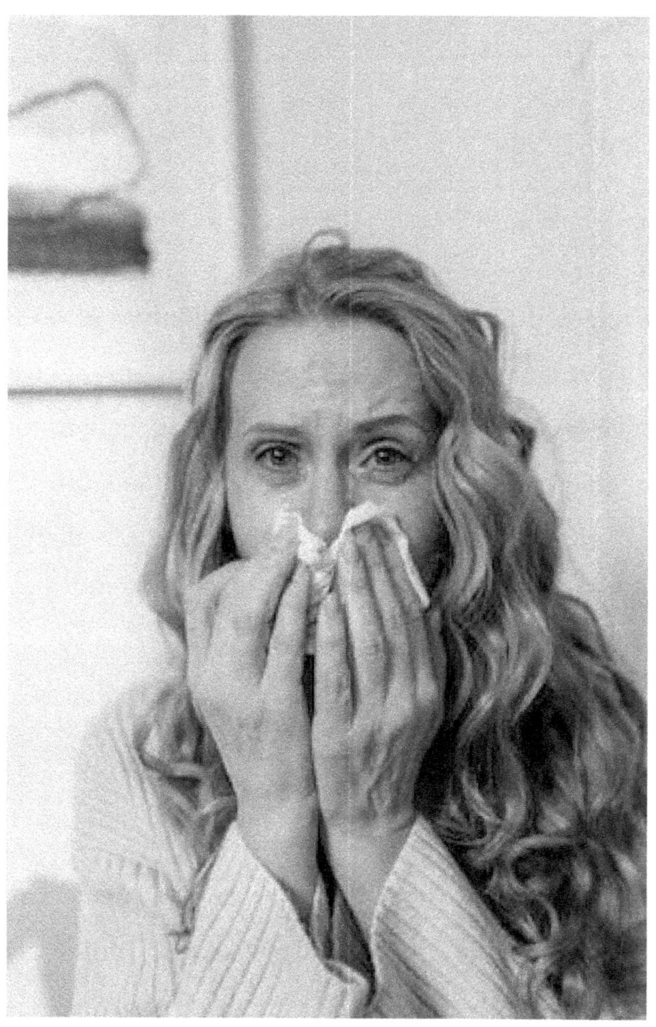

# CHAPTER 5

## CONCLUSION

Congratulations on finishing this journey towards understanding and conquering allergies. Throughout this book, we have covered the foundations of allergens, addressed common myths, and offered practical strategies to manage and reduce allergy symptoms.

## <u>Major Takeaways</u>

1.  Allergies are a consequence of an overactive immune system responding to ordinarily innocuous chemicals known as allergens.

2.  Common forms of allergies include respiratory allergies (hay fever, asthma),

food allergies, skin allergies (contact dermatitis), and insect sting allergies.

3.  It is crucial to refute misunderstandings regarding allergies, such as thinking them trivial annoyances or presuming they may be outgrown.

4.  Identifying allergy triggers is key for optimal therapy. Environmental allergies, dietary allergens, medicines, and insect allergens are frequent triggers to consider.

5.  Allergy testing procedures, such as skin prick tests and blood tests, may assist identify particular allergens that impact you.

6.  Hidden allergy causes, such as cross-reactivity and rare triggers, should be taken into consideration while treating allergies.

7. Practical ways to overcome allergies entail a multi-faceted strategy, including medicine, allergen avoidance, allergy-proofing your surroundings, and contemplating allergy immunotherapy.

8. Lifestyle modifications, such as maintaining a nutritious diet, keeping indoor air clean, reducing stress, and exercising properly, help improve allergy symptoms.

9. Strengthening the immune system with balanced diet, regular exercise, adequate sleep, and stress management may assist allergy treatment.

By following these tactics and integrating them into your everyday life, you may take control of your allergies and enjoy relief from symptoms that may have previously impaired your well-being.

Remember, it's vital to contact with healthcare specialists, such as allergists or immunologists, for individualized counseling and treatment choices depending on your unique allergies.

As you continue your journey, be updated about new research, medication choices, and lifestyle changes that may further optimize your allergy control.

Thank you for joining us on this examination of allergens. May your newfound knowledge encourage you to battle allergies and live a life free from their limits.

# APPENDIX

## Resources and Additional Information

To help you further in your path to conquer allergies, I have gathered a list of resources and supplementary information. These resources may give helpful insights, recommendations, and guidance:

**Allergy & Asthma Foundation:**

**Website: www.aafa.org**

This organization offers extensive information about allergies, asthma, and associated illnesses, including articles, instructional tools, and resources for sufferers.

American Academy of Allergy, Asthma & Immunology:

**<u>Website: www.aaaai.org</u>**

The AAAAI delivers trustworthy information about allergies, asthma, and immunology, including patient resources, research updates, and a directory to identify allergists in your region.

National Institute of Allergy and Infectious Diseases (NIAID):

**<u>Website: www.niaid.nih.gov</u>**

NIAID conducts and supports research to better understand, prevent, and treat allergies and immunologic disorders. Their website contains tools, papers, and clinical trial information.

# Allergy Support Forums and Online Communities

Participating in online groups and forums may link you with folks who have similar experiences and give support and guidance. Examples include:

1. Allergic Living Forum (www.allergicliving.com/forum) and
2. MedHelp Allergy Community (www.medhelp.org/forums/Allergy/show/127).

Remember, although these resources might be useful, always consult with trained healthcare experts for customized counsel and medical advice.

Thank you for joining me on this adventure. I wish you luck in conquering your allergies and enjoying a better, happier life.